Zero Point Healers

What Is Wrong With Me?

Holistic Health at its Best

Robert Rodgers PhD
2/14/2015

What is Wrong with Me?

Contents

© Zero Point Healers

What is Wrong with Me?

Introduction

I have experienced a wide variety of therapies over the past decade with the intention of bringing my body back into balance and harmony. Each therapy I have pursued has been useful to one extent or another – some more so than others. I am well aware that what may be helpful to someone else may not necessarily be helpful to me.

The therapies I experienced at the one end of the range were prescription medications (with side effects) to natural, holistic therapies (with few or no side effects) at the other end. My experiences with a multitude of therapies have revealed two important insights.

First, no single therapy has succeeded in reversing all of my symptoms whether they were rashes, low energy or hearing problems. Multiple therapies have always been necessary. Some were pursued at the same time. Others had to be pursued sequentially, one after the other. The body requires time and a gentle approach to come back into balance.

Second, I have concluded that Bioenergetic Assessments have been one particularly useful approach for identifying and treating symptoms of one type or another. This

What is Wrong with Me?

booklet provides a detailed explanation of Bioenergetic Assessments based on my research and personal experience. It is an approach to healing that very few people know about even though the technology was originally discovered and developed over fifty years ago. Getting the assessments is not the only reason I am healthy today. But, I credit them for giving my body a jump start to recovery over the years when I needed it most.

Robert Rodgers PhD
Zero Point Healers
www.zeropointhealers.com
Olympia, Washington

What is Wrong with Me?

The Problem in a Nutshell

When bodily discomforts flare and symptoms begin to interfere with daily activities, everyone wants to know what in the world is happening to them. A long list of unanswered questions haunts us:

- *What is causing the problem I am having?*
- *Do I have a disease?*
- *If I do have a disease, what is it?*
- *Will this problem get worse?*
- *Can the problem be treated successfully?*
- *Do I need to be seriously worried?*
- *Is something horrible happening to me?*
- *If I simply wait it out, will the symptoms eventually vanish? This has happened before. Maybe I will be lucky and be well again soon without doing anything.*
- *What in the world is wrong here?*
- *Is the problem life threatening?*

What is Wrong?

These questions are certainly familiar to everyone. We have all asked them at one point or another in our lifetime. We all want to know what is wrong with our body when we do not feel well.

What is Wrong with Me?

- *How can I get the answers to these questions now?*
- *How can I know what is really wrong with my body?*
- *Why is my body not working properly?*
- *Why am I ill?*
- *Why do I feel lousy all the time?*

No one escapes from having to face the puzzle of a body that seems to be breaking down.

Now that the questions have been asked, two approaches can be used to get answers. The first approach is a familiar one to everyone. It involves medical diagnostic testing ordered by a medical doctor. The second approach is unfamiliar to most people. It involves a generalized assessment to identify the sources of imbalances in the body. This approach is usually done by a naturopathic doctor. The medical approach is specific. The assessment approach is more general and holistic in character.

One way of distinguishing the two approaches is to think of medical diagnostic testing as a targeted approach that is initiated and interpreted by a medical doctor. Targeted diagnostic testing typically examines a narrow slice of the body's full complexity. The doctor has a hunch about a possible diagnosis and is searching for confirmation that the hunch is correct.

What is Wrong with Me?

Holistic assessments on the other hand capture the frequencies emitted by the various systems, organs, tissues and cells in the body. Some of the frequencies that are detected lie within expected parameters. Others reflect a condition that is out of range or abnormal.

Comprehensive assessments take a big picture view of the body. They are not motivated by the need to diagnose a condition. That is to say, they are not dictated by whether a doctor suspects a person has cancer or diabetes or high blood pressure and thus are not diagnostic in character.

Assessments entertain the likelihood that multiple systems in the body are compromised when symptoms are present. They open the door to reading and interpreting all of the frequencies that are emitted by the body.

I will first preview the approach taken with diagnostic medical testing. This discussion is brief. Why? Most people have firsthand experience with it. Then, I will provide a discussion of holistic assessments, the alternative approach to diagnostic testing that is unfamiliar to most people.

Medical Diagnostic Testing

Appointments with medical doctors are made when we feel lousy and experience unwanted symptoms. The doctor always wants to know why we have come. We

What is Wrong with Me?

answer the question by listing and describing our symptoms.

If the initial appointment is with an internist or family practitioner, we are referred to a specialist. For example, if the problem is a lump on our breast, we are referred to an oncologist. If the problem is a tremor, we are referred to a neurologist. There are many medical specialties. A referral could be made to any one of a large number of medical practitioners who are all specialists in treating specific symptoms of one type or another.

The oncologist evaluates tumors for cancer. If the test is positive, they cut it out, blast it with radiation or saturate it with chemotherapy. If the problem is a tremor, a neurologist evaluates the patient for one among a number of neurological conditions such as Parkinson's disease or Lou Gehrig's disease (ALS). Once a diagnosis is tendered, specific treatments in the form of medicines or surgeries are recommended. In both examples a doctor assigns a diagnosis.

Depending on the specialty, medical tests are ordered to support a diagnosis. The tests may include blood tests, x-rays, biopsies, or various scans of the body using Magnetic Resonance Imaging (MRIs), Pet Scans or Computerized Tomography (CT Scans). These tests are specific in character. The doctor specifies which tests (out of hundreds of possibilities) that should be done for a diagnosis to be confirmed or disconfirmed. The type of test requested depends on what the doctor is looking for: Is it a deficiency in calcium or an abundance of toxins of one type or another of ...? In other words, the doctor has a narrowly defined question that needs to be answered.

Results of initial tests are often negative. That is to say, they do not show anything is abnormal or out of range. A mystery remains about what is wrong. The doctor reevaluates the situation and usually orders more tests to see if a definitive diagnosis can be confirmed. They might even change their original hunch about the disease. It is not uncommon for the cost of tests to run into the tens (if not hundreds) of thousands of dollars.

Sometimes, definitive answers are revealed. For example, we may learn that we have a calcium deficiency or that there is an abundance of cancer cells in the blood. Such results direct the doctor to prescribe specific therapies that are intended to treat the symptoms.

In summary, targeted diagnostic testing involves the examination of a specific inquiry which relates to a narrowly defined issue in the body. For example ophthalmologists only consider potential problems involving the eyes, not the bladder. There may be something seriously wrong with the bladder but an ophthalmologist will never detect the problem. They are not looking for it.

Likewise, the urologist will never consider problems with eyes. They focus on identifying problems with the bladder. The bladder may be fine but there could be serious problems with the eyes. The urologist will never see it because they are not looking for it. The urologist knows nothing about eyes. The ophthalmologist knows nothing about bladders.

Employed as a professor for 20 years I had the benefit of receiving free medical care from the university medical center. Whenever any problem emerged, I routinely made an appointment with a medical doctor for free medical assistance. Why not?

At one point I began having an extensive rash all over my legs and chest. To take advantage of my free health benefit, I made an appointment with an allergy specialist at the medical center. The doctor ordered a long series of blood tests that considered many possibilities - from infections to cancer. The lab took more blood out of my body than I thought possible.

At my follow-up appointment I was told all tests were negative. The doctor did not know what was causing my rash. She ordered a steroid cream which was formulated

What is Wrong with Me?

to treat my symptoms (the rash). The rash disappeared as long as I applied the cream. When I stopped using it, the rash returned. It had spread.

Medical tests are ordered to answer a specific question. There are very precise tests that measure the level of hormones such as dopamine, serotonin and adrenaline. There are specialized medical tests that measure the quantity of specific vitamins and minerals in the body. There are comprehensive medical tests that assess the health of specific organs like the liver and kidneys. And so forth and so on. All such tests are of course excellent, but they offer only a piecemeal story.

In summary, medical diagnostic testing focuses on a specific question. It is often the case that only one system in the body is tested (either a lung or a heart or a colon for example). Information revealed from the diagnostic test will always be constrained by the question that is posed. In the case of the problem with my rash, tests provided no information that would inform a diagnosis other than the fact I had a rash (which I knew before I saw the doctor).

What is Wrong with Me?

Comprehensive Assessments

The type of comprehensive, holistic assessment I have become familiar with is known as a Bioenergetic Assessment. Physicians who do Bioenergetic Assessments for their patients are usually naturopath doctors though some medical doctors do them as well.

What is the difference between the approach taken by a medical doctor and that of a naturopath doctor? As a general rule, naturopaths focus their diagnostic inquiries to identify reasons why symptoms exist. Medical doctors on the other hand focus on the treatment of symptoms. Medical doctors are much like the defense on a football team. They prevent "attacks" from causing troublesome problems. Naturopaths are interested in identifying the root cause of illness. They are much like the offensive unit of a football team. Naturopaths focus on the processes in the body that can potentially make the situation worse.

The idea behind Bioenergetic Assessments is to identify all of the frequencies that are emitted by the body. Testing is done by a computer analysis of one form or another. The analysis generated by Bioenergetic assessments identifies imbalances and problems that are currently present in the body.

Various technologies that use Bioenergetic principles exist. Some assess the disturbances in meridians in the

What is Wrong with Me?

body using tiny electrical impulses that are sent through acupuncture points located on the hands and feet. The form of Bioenergetic testing I will preview in more detail involves analysis of imbalances using a sample of saliva.

A computer-based Bioenergetic Assessment measures the integrity of every system in the body. Imbalances are identified that can be caused by allergies, infections, yeast, mold, chemicals, heavy metals and other toxic exposures. The test instrument is capable of performing over 17,000 individual assessments.

- Is there an infection in the right upper molar? The Bioenergetic Assessment will find it.
- Is there an overabundance of iron in the body? The Bioenergetic Assessment will find it.
- Is a staph or strep infection present? The Bioenergetic Assessment will find it.

Really? How is this possible? How are such problems revealed without being specifically targeted?

Bioenergetic Assessments identify the frequencies that are currently emitted by the various organs and tissues of the body as revealed from analysis of the saliva. Just as with medical diagnostic testing, some of the frequencies found are well within the normal range. For example, frequencies associated with the normal function of the heart may be present or absent as the case may be. If the cardiac function is compromised, testing will pick up the problem.

A good analogy to the Bioenergetic Assessment approach is how we tune into a radio station. Everyone is familiar with the different frequencies of radio stations. Shift the dial on the radio to the right or left and we connect to a different radio station that is broadcasting on its authorized frequency. If you do not set the dial squarely on the station frequency you wish to hear, you will hear static. To hear the station clearly you have to set the dial to the precise frequency that is broadcast by the radio station.

Frequencies emitted by the body work in a similar fashion. Each heavy metal emits a unique frequency. Iron emits a frequency that is different from the frequency of manganese. Similarly, each bacteria (and there and hundreds) and each virus (and there are hundreds) emits its own unique frequency. All chemicals, organs, substances and tissues in the body emit their own unique frequency signal.

If the frequency falls out of the normal range, Bioenergetic Assessments can spot organs that are compromised. It also finds the presence of toxins, bacteria and even electromagnetic pollution that has compromised the ability of the body to function normally. This is possible because everything has a unique frequency signal.

What is Wrong with Me?

In summary, there is no preconceived idea of what will be revealed with Bioenergetic Assessments. The test asks the body what is up by analyzing the frequencies from saliva samples. The body answers through the myriad of frequency signal stamps. The analysis is performed using a sophisticated computer program that is orchestrated by a trained practitioner.

What is the Difference between Bioenergetic Assessments and Diagnostic Medical Tests?

Hear Dr. Ivy Faber Answer This Question at:

http://www.blog.parkinsonsrecovery.com/difference-bioenergetic-testing-standard-medical-test/

There is really nothing like a Bioenergetic Assessment. It assesses all systems in the body and yields a comprehensive picture of what is within the normal range and what is not. It utilizes the autonomic energy system of the body to identify the root causes of dis-ease. Once identified, remedies to bring the body back into balance are identified.

Bioenergetic Assessments are not a quick fix. Results depend on a variety of factors including the number and penetration of toxins in the body as well as the health of the detox pathways including the kidneys, colon and liver.

© Zero Point Healers

What is Wrong with Me?

In contrast, the medical tests are used to confirm or disconfirm a diagnosis. They are not used to pinpoint the cause(s) of the problem. Many of the tests use a sample of blood. Toxins can pass through the blood stream quickly before they find a home in the tissues of the body to hang out. Blood tests will usually not reveal the presence of most toxins unless the exposure is very recent. Blood tests in most cases do not detect the exposure to toxins from long ago.

Bioenergetic Assessments have the capability of detecting the probable cause of imbalances which may have origins recently or long ago - perhaps last month or as early as birth or childhood. They do not analyze a sample of blood.

Since most people are interested in getting relief from symptoms, the focus of medical tests is to diagnose the present condition so that symptoms can be suppressed. In some cases relief can be experienced relatively quickly. Appropriate medications can produce relatively fast symptomatic relief (assuming side effects are not problematic) though the cause remains. In contrast, quick results are seldom seen with the protocols indicated from Bioenergetic Assessments. They are designed to detect the cause of symptoms and identify therapies that help bring the body back into balance again.

What is Wrong with Me?

In a more general sense diagnostic testing is driven by the need for a diagnosis. It is targeted. Bioenergetic Assessments are comprehensive. There is no preconceived idea of what will be discovered. The differences are summarized in the table below.

Table 1. Comparison of Diagnostic Medical Testing with Bioenergetic Assessments

Diagnostic Medical Testing	Bioenergetic Assessments
Doctor has a diagnostic hunch. Specific medical tests are ordered to confirm the diagnosis.	Doctor asks the body what is wrong. The body answers by the frequencies it emits
Results of tests are often negative indicating nothing is wrong.	Testing reveals sources of imbalances.
Testing is costly, often running into tens of thousands of dollars, but is covered by health insurance.	Testing is relatively inexpensive but is not covered by most health insurance plans.
Testing may not necessarily reveal presence of bacterial or viral infections, toxins or allergies.	Testing reveals presence of infections, toxins and food sensitivities.
Purpose of testing is to confirm a diagnosis.	Purpose of testing is to identify the causes of symptoms
A series of diagnostic tests may be necessary to diagnose a condition.	One comprehensive assessment is done. Follow-up assessments are done after treatment.

What is Wrong with Me?

Overview of Bioenergetic Assessments

There is now a critical body of health care practitioners who have acquired the necessary computer technology and have been trained to perform Bioenergetic Assessments. The naturopath doctor who has done assessments for me over the past ten years is Ivy Faber, ND. Her clinic is located in Canton, Georgia. Ivy is a gifted doctor who brings to the table three decades of experience working with patients with a variety of chronic illnesses. I chose her initially because she does long distance assessments for people. I have never actually met her in person.

Dr. Faber has now run eight Bioenergetic Assessments for me as her patient. Results of each assessment have been invaluable. Directed by her competent guidance and skill, the root cause of one symptom or another has been identified and treated successfully. Bioenergetic Assessments she ran for me also provided early signals of illnesses that were in the making, but had not yet manifested as troublesome symptoms.

Not one of the assessment reports I received diagnosed a disease. I was never informed that I had "chronic fatigue

17

What is Wrong with Me?

illness" or "autoimmune disease" or "cancer" or "Lupus."
As noted, assessments do not diagnose.

This suits my preference and requirements for medical
care to a tea. I have no interest in having any such labels
attached to my psyche. There is no doubt in my mind that
a diagnosis of any disease is simply an educated guess by a
qualified medical doctor. Even if a diagnosis is correct, I
personally do not want to identify with it or hold it in my
consciousness. Any diagnosis, whatever the name, is
inevitably associated with the energy of doom and gloom.
Many diseases are declared to be irreversible and
degenerative. If I think I have little chance of reversing my
symptoms, I have little chance of reversing them.

My own research on chronic illnesses – and Parkinson's
disease in particular – has revealed that many people are
misdiagnosed. A broken bone can be diagnosed with
almost perfect accuracy, but there is no definitive way to
pinpoint an accurate diagnosis for many conditions,
especially Parkinson's. A diagnosis is the opinion of one
person which is why many people seek a second opinion.
Unfortunately, many people take a diagnosis as fact.

Speaking as a researcher, I have concluded that when
symptoms begin to interfere with the lifestyle of a person,
many systems in the body are impacted. If the kidneys and
colon are not functioning at their peak capacity (as is the

case for many people) there will be a critical excess of toxins that are trapped in the tissues of the body. All organs will be affected. The liver is the major detox organ of the body which is why it is so large. Everyone's liver is compromised to one extent or another. If the damage is excessive, toxins will build up in the tissues of the body.

If you need to have a designation of a disease for your symptoms, do not bother exploring the Bioenergetic Assessment computer technology. This is not the information that you will get from a Bioenergetic Assessment. Assessments are holistic. They scan all systems in the body. Medical doctors diagnose a condition. Although I do not wish to have a label attached to my symptoms, you may. The preferred resource for you would be a medical doctor, or MD.

What is a Bioenergetic Computer Assessment?

Hear Dr. Ivy Faber Answer This Question
http://www.blog.parkinsonsrecovery.com/bioenergetic-assessment/

Bioenergetic Assessments utilize sophisticated computer software that measure and evaluate the energetic balance of all systems in the body. The assessment focuses on each person's individual needs. It does this by tapping into the autonomic energy system of the patient's body. The framework for assessments was developed by the Chinese thousands of years ago.

Something has caused the body to be out of balance. What is it? Bioenergetic Assessments focus on the cause(s) of imbalances in the body that happen to be expressed in the form of symptoms. Once the causes have been identified, appropriate remedies are recommended to help the body come back into balance. Many remedies that are used are homeopathic in character. Homeopathy is a 'tried and true' approach for helping the body to heal itself.

The computer testing used by Dr. Faber is based on a sample of the patient's saliva. Results provide a highly accurate method of determining prioritive energetic imbalances in the body. It is through analysis and evaluation of the bio-chemistry of saliva that the causes of imbalances are identified. These findings are used to identify the remedies that are needed to correct the imbalances.

Bioenergetic Assessments evaluate scenarios involving detoxification, nutritional support, glandular support, hormone imbalances, genetic predispositions, allergies and emotional issues. Imbalances can be caused by any number of factors including allergies, infections, yeast and mold overgrowth, chemicals, heavy metals and a host of other toxins. The assessment automatically reveals which natural nutrients, vitamins, homeopathic remedies, herbs or other treatments the body needs for a return to a healthy, balanced condition.

This "wave of the future" assessment makes it possible to identify all systems and organs in the body that have been compromised. The intent of assessments is to restore systems of the body that have been compromised to their normal function.

Bioenergetic Assessments are intended for investigational purposes only. They have not been evaluated by the U.S. Food and Drug Administration. It is intended for investigational use only and is not meant for formal medical diagnosis.

Bioenergetic Assessments are Holistic

Bioenergetic Assessments consider the whole picture. They take into consideration all systems and organs in the body. From my own personal experience with them, the assessment also pinpoints future problem areas. This means you can correct the imbalances before more symptoms surface. Having the results in hand is a great motivator to give your body what it needs the correct any and all imbalances.

What is Wrong with Me?

- **Bioenergetic Assessments are safe.** – Assessments are based on a saliva sample. No needle pricks, blood samples or biopsies are required.

- **Bioenergetic Assessments consider the interrelated health of all systems in the body** –The functions of all systems in the body are analyzed, revealing areas that need attention.

- **Bioenergetic Assessments are affordable** – When compared to the cost of standard medical tests, the cost of the assessments is affordable though they are not typically covered by health insurance.

- **Bioenergetic Assessments identify ways to enhance the viability of all systems in the body** – The focus is on strengthening all systems and organs in the body so that healing can occur naturally. The emphasis is not on disease. Rather, it is focused on wellness.

- **Bioenergetic Assessments provide detailed information about problem areas** – Results are specific, indicating the names of specific heavy metals and other toxins that are present as well as the names of bacteria and pathogens that have contaminated the tissues and organs of the body.

© Zero Point Healers

What is Wrong with Me?

Specifics are also suggested with regard to foods that induce allergic reactions.

- **Bioenergetic Assessments inform specific recommendations for therapeutic interventions –** Because the assessment is specific, therapies are identified and recommended that are individualized rather than taking a more general, hit and miss approach to treatment.

- **Bioenergetic Assessments are reliable and valid–** Bioenergetic Assessment technology was developed a half century ago. Use of the technology has helped countless thousands restore their health. Considerable evidence is now available on its reliability and validity.

- **Bioenergetic Assessments identify future problem areas that may have yet to materialize –** Assessments catch problems that patients may not even be aware of because they are at the initial stage of development. Symptoms will not be experienced until a problem becomes more acute. It takes time for symptoms to show up. Correcting the problem in its early stages is much easier than correcting it when a symptom becomes acute. It makes sense to correct a problem before symptoms are experienced.

What is Wrong with Me?

- **Bioenergetic Assessments prioritize problem areas** – Although all issues of imbalance are identified by the assessment, problems that merit immediate attention are highlighted. This informs therapeutic interventions that are urgently needed and treatments that can be placed on hold for later treatment. The body cannot heal all imbalances with a one shot treatment.

Summary of Bioenergetic Assessment Benefits

There are many different tests that provide useful information about the causes of imbalances in your body. Computerized Bioenergetic Assessments are approach that offers an impressive array of benefits. They are:

- *Safe*

- *Noninvasive*

- *Affordable*

- *Comprehensive*

The assessments offer a snapshot analysis of all systems and organs in the body. Findings are specific as to causes of problems. Recommended therapies are individually tailored to address the most acute issues. Because the

What is Wrong with Me?

body is not bombarded with too many treatments at the same time, healing unfolds gently.

What is Special about a Bioenergetic Assessment?
Hear Dr. Ivy Faber Answer This Question at:

http://www.blog.parkinsonsrecovery.com/special-bioenergetic-assessment

Until development of Bioenergetic Assessments it was not possible to evaluate the overall function of all systems and organs in the body. The Bioenergetics Assessment is revolutionary in that it takes into consideration the full spectrum of imbalances in the body without having to cut open the body with surgery to see what is inside. Bioenergetic Assessments identify:

- *Specific organs that are struggling to function at peak capacity.*
- *Substances that have compromised the efficiency of elimination organs including the kidneys, liver and colon.*
- *Disease states that have been "percolating" in their early stages before they have been manifested as symptoms.*

What is Wrong with Me?

What Will You Receive When You Order an Assessment?

Different doctors will likely proceed differently when doing an assessment for you. I will describe the procedure Dr. Faber uses. Several days after ordering my Bioenergetic Assessment I receive a snail mail correspondence from Harmony Health in the mail that contains a vial. Instructions in this mailing indicate you must fill 1/4 of the vial with your own saliva the first thing in the morning after getting up, making sure that your palate and mouth are clear of food particles. I then mail the saliva sample to Dr. Ivy Faber, ND at Harmony Health in Canton, Georgia using a priority US postal service.

Once the sample is received by Harmony Health, the computerized assessment is run and analyzed personally by Dr. Faber. When the assessment has been completed, you will receive a written report of findings in the mail. The report includes a complete listing of specific infections and toxins that have been identified in addition to a listing of suspected food sensitivities. Specific recommendations are offered for how all imbalances can be rectified with natural herbs, cleanses, homeopathic treatments or other treatment modalities.

The written report of findings is followed up with a personal phone consultation with Dr. Faber. During the call she discusses the findings and answers your questions. She also explains how the various imbalances can potentially be rectified with the treatments she has recommended.

Bioenergetic Assessments offer important clues about where the real problems lie. The sooner you identify the cause of your symptoms and launch a program to address them, the sooner you will have the opportunity to reverse symptoms.

If, for example, you happened to have been diagnosed with a cancerous tumor, the tumor is a symptom. The cause may be due to a feeble circulation system that allows the cancerous cells to form into fibroid globules. You can have your doctor remove the tumor surgically, but if the problem is one of poor circulation, other tumors will pop out in other parts of the body. This happens to people all the time. Causes have to be rectified for the problem to be solved.

The Bioenergetics Assessment approach that has worked for me is straightforward.

What is Wrong with Me?

1. Identify the imbalances in your body.
2. Get a consultation from a knowledgeable doctor.
3. Start treatments that address the source of the imbalances.
4. Do not expect symptoms will disappear with a single treatment. The body can heal itself, but authentic healing is seldom quick. If you want to believe you are better, simply treat the symptoms and forget about what is causing them.

How Much Do Bioenergetic Assessments Cost?

Obviously the cost of an assessment and the recommended treatments will depend on the physician who does the assessment and the cost of recommended treatments. There are many naturopath doctors now who provide this service. It is likely you can locate a naturopath in your area who can provide a Bioenergetic Assessment and consultation for you. Dr. Faber offers long distance consultations.

My experience of course is with Dr. Faber who did not become a naturopath to become wealthy. She practices medicine to help people get their lives back. The cost of her assessments are, in my view, a bargain, especially when you compare it to the cost of standard medical tests and traditional medical treatments .

What is Wrong with Me?

As noted, her assessments include a comprehensive written report of the assessment, a phone consultation with her personally and detailed recommendations for treatments. Services of other physicians may vary depending on whether they offer phone consultations.

Insights from a Decade of Experience

By way of further explanation, I want to discuss my personal experience with getting a series of eight Bioenergetic Assessments over the past ten years. As a companion to my discussion, listen to the phone consultation I had with Dr. Faber about my most recent results. Taken together you will have a rich understanding about the scope and detail of the information and recommendations that are generated from the assessment itself. What have I discovered from getting eight Bioenergetic Assessments over the past ten years?

Hear Dr. Ivy Faber provide a consultation for an Assessment done for me at:

http://www.blog.parkinsonsrecovery.com/example-bioenergetic-assessment/

The recommended treatments helped to restore my life force when my energy was depleted and identified the probable cause of symptoms that I happened to

What is Wrong with Me?

experience at the time of each assessment. Each of the eight assessments have provided information and treatment protocols that have been immensely valuable were "dead on" target. I say this because the findings revealed the causal reasons for long standing problems. Some started in my childhood.

The detail included in each assessment is unbelievable. An assessment of the health of organs is provided, as is the presence of harmful toxic substances and bacteria. It is even possible for an assessment to target a specific tooth that has a chronic and life threatening infection.

I have no chronic health issues today. This is due in in part to therapies that successfully addressed the imbalances that were identified in the assessments. I believe the therapies that were recommended in the assessments have been instrumental to my success with maintaining excellent health. They have not however been the sole therapy that I have pursued over the years.

Bioenergetic Assessments are not a quick fix, nor are they an easy solution to chronic health conditions. Assessments help reveal the root cause of symptoms. The immune system may be compromised. If so, it is not resilient enough initially to handle any treatment that targets a root cause of an illness. For most people – myself included – organs needed for a successful detox program are

© Zero Point Healers

already compromised. The organs that are needed to eliminate the toxins and other harmful critters must be gently nudged back into balance if any treatment protocol is to be successful in addressing the problems. When the kidneys, colon and liver become more functional and are "back on line" so to speak, treatments can be initiated that directly focus on healing the root cause of symptoms.

Any attempt to "heal" everything that is out of balance all at once will result in a virtual freezing of the body. The body can only do so much work at a time. Freezing is similar to what happens when a computer freezes and shuts down. It will still work, but some of the programs have been temporarily disabled.

A single Bioenergetic Assessment with its concomitant treatment protocol rarely results in a magical "cure" or "quick fix". If a condition is chronic, it has likely taken years for symptoms to emerge. It makes perfect sense to me that the body needs time to reverse imbalances that have been in the making for years.

My personal experience has been that authentic healing from the inside–out inevitably takes time and patience. The body needs time to bring all systems in the body back into balance. You can heal most headaches with an aspirin, but the headaches will return unless the underlying cause is found and addressed.

What is Wrong with Me?

Patience and persistence are needed if you are serious about supporting your body's ability to return to health and wellness. Explore other treatment options if you expect to get quick results. Prescription medicine protocols do sometimes offer quick results. There are always risks however. The side effects of the medications may be worse than the positive outcome of the treatment. Also troubling is the reality that when a patient stops taking prescription medications, symptoms will almost always return in most cases. Why? The cause of the problem has not been found and addressed.

My personal preference is the assessment approach. It offers the opportunity to explore the root causes of symptoms. Many people falsely belief that a single cause is at play. My experience over the years is that many causal factors work in concert to manifest the symptoms that are experienced. Treating a single factor opens the door to seeing what else needs to be healed.

Authentic healing is much like peeling an onion. Think of each layer of the onion as a cause of your symptoms. As one layer of the union is pealed, the next layer is revealed. Once that layer is healed, it can also be pealed. The next layer (or cause) is presented to be healed.

If you are lucky, multiple causes will be resolved with a single treatment protocol. My experience has been that each causal factor must be addressed one by one. Each new Bioenergetic Assessment uses the most recent saliva sample, revealing new issues that need to be addressed. Our bodies are intricate and complicated. To heal they need gentle interventions and a barrel full of patience peppered with trust that the body really does know how to heal itself.

One of the most fascinating aspects of Bioenergetic Assessments is that each report is different. Initial assessments reveal the problems that are the most acute. Once these initial problems are resolved, the next assessment reveals the next layer of issues that need to be addressed. The body has an uncanny way of communicating what is needed next.

Example of a Bioenergetic Assessment and Recommended Treatment Protocol

To explain more precisely what a bioenergetics assessment entails, I will now provide the nitty gritty details from my most recent assessment. In so doing, you will get a detailed preview of exactly what can be discovered from an assessment. Obviously, the specifics of my personal situation will be of little interest to anyone but me, but taking a closer look at what an assessment

What is Wrong with Me?

entails will help you understand what a bioenergetics does for the patient.

I am in my late sixties and have no health problems thanks, in part, to the Bioenergetic Assessment technology. The naturopath doctor who ran my most recent assessment is Dr. Ivy Faber. I have never met Dr. Faber in person. All of the assessments were done using snail mail, emails and phone consultations.

My most recent Bioenergetics Assessment identified organs that were in need of support and systems in my body that were compromised. My explanation below will detail the findings and recommended treatments. Dr. Faber recommended a treatment protocol that was developed using her extensive experience working with hundreds of patients with a wide variety of chronic and debilitating illnesses. I followed the protocol she recommended.

Step by Step Description of Bioenergetic Assessments

Recall that your health care provider (Dr. Faber in my case) will need to get a saliva sample from you and a list of your symptoms. Dr. Faber sends her patients a vial to deposit your saliva (spit) and a general health questionnaire. Both the saliva sample and health history are mailed back to her using priority mail.

What is Wrong with Me?

Symptoms I reported for my most recent assessment were:

- Hair loss
- Frequent urination
- Tinnitus
- Difficulty swallowing pills

All of these symptoms were not acute (i.e., recent). They were chronic in the sense that I have struggled with them for many years. Clearly, I do not have the expectation that these symptoms will be completely reversed after taking a single treatment protocol.

Bioenergetic Assessments are done by a trained practitioner who may have to spend hours figuring out what therapies will offer the best chance of nudging the body back into balance. Frequencies from your saliva sample are not simply read by the computer program and a resultant result automatically produced. Nothing is automatic or mechanical about doing the Bioenergetic Assessment.

Dr. Faber is the first to acknowledge that running the assessment takes extensive training and experience. She runs all of the assessments herself. Some of the assessments she has done have taken her anywhere from two to four hours for her to complete. Others take less time.

Results of a Bioenergetic Assessment

My most recent assessment revealed the presence of the following heavy metal toxins:

- Methyl (organic mercury salt)
- Mercury
- Niccolum
- Aluminum

Dr. Ivy explained during my consultation that these heavy metals were the root cause of my symptoms. Once I get these toxins out of my body, the symptoms should evidence of relief.

It is not an easy to excrete or otherwise remove these nasty heavy metals from the tissues of my body. Why? Dr. Faber explained that heavy metals were literally glued to my tissues. To be successful, the treatments have to soften up the "glue" so to speak in order for the heavy metals to detach from the tissues and organs. I obviously can't put my body in a hot oven to soften up the "glue". The detachment process takes time. The heavy metal toxins identified from the analysis of my saliva have occupied my

What is Wrong with Me?

body for decades. I know this because most of my symptoms appeared years ago.

The eloquence of the assessment is that there is a match of treatments that are compatible with the specific frequencies of my body. Many possible treatments can be used to detox heavy metals. What specific treatment is right for my body? I have obviously chased after many detox protocols. While they all have helped to one extent or another over the years, no detox treatment protocol has obviously succeeded in eliminating the heavy metals from my body that have been causing the symptoms.

The written assessment included the detox protocol that Dr. Faber recommended. She listed three homeopathic remedies: one for heavy metals, one for assisting drainage and tonification of the kidneys and one for clarifying disturbances in the lymph matrix. She also prescribed a product containing chlorella and a comprehensive liver detox.

Results of the Treatments

I am now half way through taking the treatments Dr. Faber prescribed. Results are encouraging. My recent experience follows the pattern of success that I have experienced with my other Bioenergetic Assessments over the years.

What is Wrong with Me?

1. My tinnitus (ringing in the ear) is better.
2. My hair growth has improved.
3. Swallowing is easier.

Best of all – a symptom I did not even report to Dr. Ivy Faber has shown improvement. Dark spots on my hands have been clearing. Discoloration of the skin and blotches at the extremities of the body – in my case the hands – are an indication of toxins. The body always deposits toxins at the extremities of the body, as far away from the vital organs as possible if they cannot otherwise be eliminated. As I watch the brown blotches on my hands disappear, I can celebrate the implication. Toxins that have lodged in my internal organs are also clearing. How cool is that?

Allergy Testing

All Bioenergetic Assessments offer the patient a listing of food sensitivities. My report indicates problems with cow milk (dairy), malt, barley, kefir, cheese, red dye number 3 and yellow dye number 6. During my detox treatments it is a good idea to avoid these foods and food additives.

Dr. Faber explained during my consultation with her that a long standing, fundamental allergy for me is any food containing dairy products. Other food sensitivities can be probably resolved when I excrete the heavy metals that are compromising the efficient function of my digestive organs. Once the heavy metals have been eliminated, my body will be better able to successfully digest these foods despite the fact my assessment currently shows I have a sensitivity to them. As a chronic food allergen, I must always avoid eating dairy or take the consequences. When I eat dairy, I will always feel horrible afterward (and always have felt horrible).

A valuable contribution of Bioenergetic Assessments is the identification of food sensitivities. Many people are accustomed to eating the same foods without realizing they make them seriously ill. Once you know which foods to avoid, you are in a position to take control of your health once again. When you stop eating the foods that are making you ill you will feel a great deal better.

In the spirit of helping you become familiar with precisely what a Bioenergetic Assessment consultation entails, the recording of my own consultation with Dr. Faber about my own assessment results follows.

My chat with Dr. Faber provides a rich perspective on how naturopath doctors help people like me (and you) to reverse our symptoms, regain energy and move back into the flow of life as it was meant to be lived.

What is Wrong with Me?

Summary

Bioenergetic Assessments are not automated or generalized. They are not the result of a routine output of a computerized program. The practitioner considers the symptoms that are being experienced against the imbalances that have been revealed. The focus is always centered on identifying the root causes of the symptoms - not on merely treating the symptoms so that temporary relief is experienced. The idea is to help the body heal so that relief is long lasting. Perpetual treatments of symptoms are thus unnecessary.

One smart way to support a return to health and wellness is to find a naturopath doctor who will run a Bioenergetic Assessment for you. You of course are very familiar with your own symptoms. Results of a Bioenergetic Assessment will offer rich insights into the cause of them. Once the cause is known treatments can be found that offer the promise of inside-out healing. You obviously do not have to pursue the treatments recommended by a Bioenergetics Assessment, but at least you have a global snapshot of where all the imbalances in your body lie. For most people who have a chronic illness, there are many.

Once you know more about the imbalances in your body and the cause of your symptoms, you can pursue therapies of one type of another that address imbalances. Instead of numbing the symptoms, you address their root cause.

The Bioenergetics Assessment report will recommend therapies that have been formulated to address the cause. Recommendations may, for example, include suggestions of supplements, homeopathic remedies or other detoxing products that will specifically address the problems that have been identified.

The reason Bioenergetic Assessments are useful is that they take into consideration the interrelationships of all systems in the body. This opens the possibility for the practitioner to identify the root causes of the symptoms.

- Does the problem reside in kidneys that are not functioning at their peak capacity?
- Is the liver seriously compromised?
- Is the digestive system clogged with toxins?
- Is the heart contaminated with strep?
- Are the lungs infested with a staph infection or candida?

Recommendations are formulated to address systems in the body that interfere with the efficient function of vital organs.

What is Wrong with Me?

Bioenergetic Assessments are not a quick fix to chronic health conditions. They must be accompanied by other healthy lifestyle habits.

1. If your diet is unhealthy, you will continue to be sick.
2. If you refuse to move your body and exercise regularly, your lymph system will be perpetually compromised.
3. If you insist on holding beliefs that are not in your best and highest good (such as "I deserve this disease"), illness will linger.

I have personally found Bioenergetic Assessments to be instrumental in my own journey to health and wellness. I recommend them to anyone, even if they are not currently experiencing a chronic health condition.

Why not experience a Bioenergetic Assessment for yourself and see what you think? It will (usually) not work any magic relief for you. In my book of truths, the result is better than treating symptoms for the rest of your life. I prefer the alternative approach.

1. Discover and treat the cause of problems.
2. Manifest health and wellness rather than perpetuate disease and illness.

© Zero Point Healers

What is Wrong with Me?

This, after all, is the value in life that have always treasured. How about you?

Bioenergetic Assessment Resource

Harmony Health
770-345-6614
Canton, Georgia
Email: info@harmonyhealthinc.com
www.**harmony**healthinc.com